❁ The ❁
WIGMAKERS

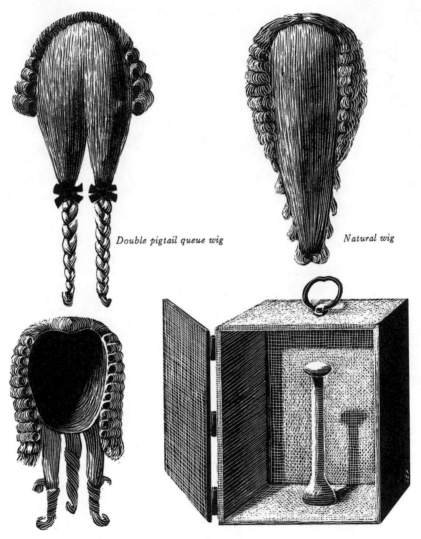

Double pigtail queue wig

Natural wig

Knotted wig

Wig box

COLONIAL AMERICAN CRAFTSMEN

The
WIGMAKERS

WRITTEN & ILLUSTRATED BY

Leonard Everett Fisher

FRANKLIN WATTS, INC.
575 Lexington Avenue, New York, N. Y. 10022

For my mother and father

SBN 531-01039-2

Library of Congress Catalog Card Number: 65-21628
© Copyright 1965 by Leonard Everett Fisher
Printed in the United States of America

4 5

Colonial Americans

THE CABINETMAKERS
THE GLASSMAKERS
THE HATTERS
THE PAPERMAKERS
THE PRINTERS
THE SCHOOLMASTERS
THE SHOEMAKERS
THE SILVERSMITHS
THE TANNERS
THE WEAVERS
THE WIGMAKERS

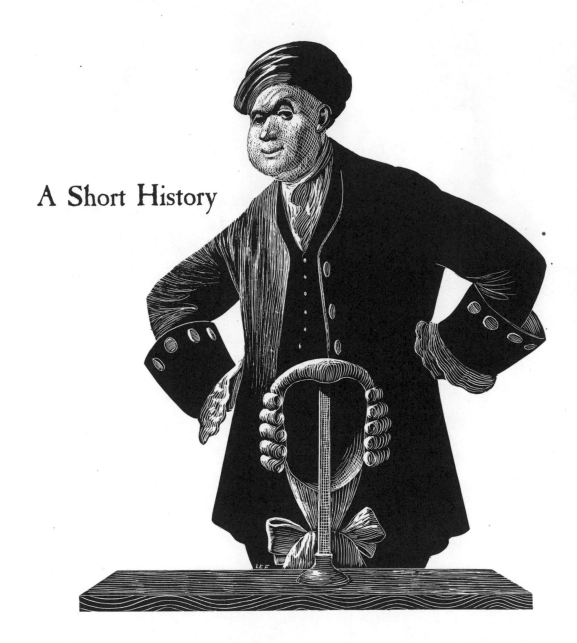

A Short History

IN THE YEAR 1624, EUROPE WAS A CHANGing, restless place. The leading powers of that unhappy continent were engaged in a painful war that was to last for thirty years in all. Germany was not one nation, but a group of quarreling cities and principalities. The Dutch were waging a desperate fight against the Spanish. Denmark had entered the war in Germany. James I, King of England, was almost at the end of his reign. In Italy the age of its most glorious art, the Renaissance, had already run its course a hundred years before.

In France, the sad and shy twenty-three-year-old King Louis XIII had entrusted the affairs of state to his chief minister, Cardinal Richelieu, and had retired to his apartments at the royal palace, the Louvre, to brood over his troubles — among them his falling hair. The young King suffered from the same untimely baldness that had plagued the royal houses of France for nine hundred years — ever since the days of Charles the Bald, grandson of Charlemagne, King of the Franks.

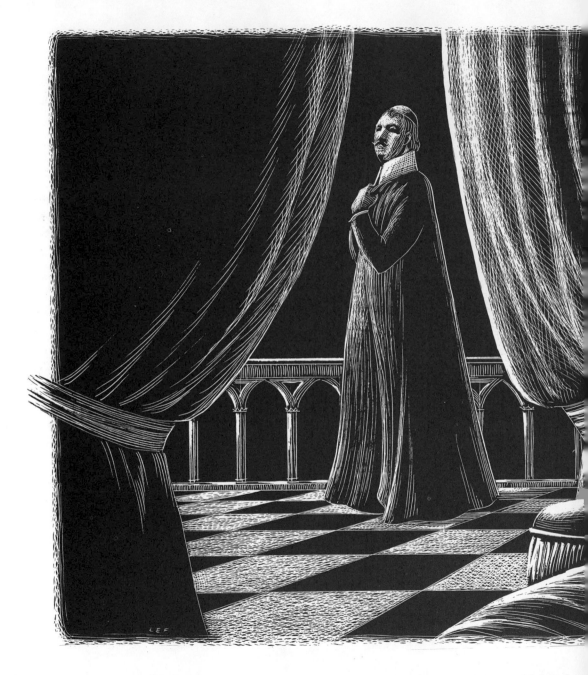

King Louis XIII of France brooded over his troubles

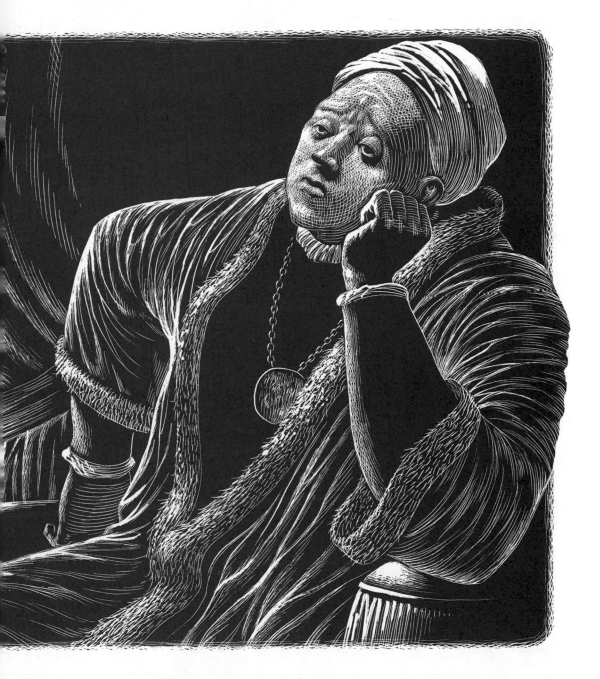

while Cardinal Richelieu attended to affairs of state   ❋ **9** ❋

Ancient Greek actors,
wearing masks, used wigs
as part of their makeup

The *HISTORY*

It was a time of great affairs, but amid them this one young man's small personal misfortune brought about a royal decision. It seemed unimportant, but it changed hairdressing fashions for the next one hundred and sixty-five years. King Louis XIII of France put on a wig. The French called it a *perruque.*

A wig, as everyone knows, is a false arrangement of hair to cover the head. Wigs had been known and used for thousands of years before Louis decided to improve his appearance. Both men and women had worn wigs in ancient Egypt, and had placed them on the heads of mummies. Ancient Greek actors had used wigs as part of their stage makeup. The highborn ladies of early Rome had worn wigs made of golden curls cut from the heads of barbarian captives. A jester in the court of Elizabeth I of England wore a wig, and Elizabeth herself is said to have had a large variety of wigs to cover her thinning hair.

Nevertheless, up to the time when Louis XIII put on his *perruque* in 1624, such head coverings had not been generally used. Now it became the fashion in France for people to wear wigs whether

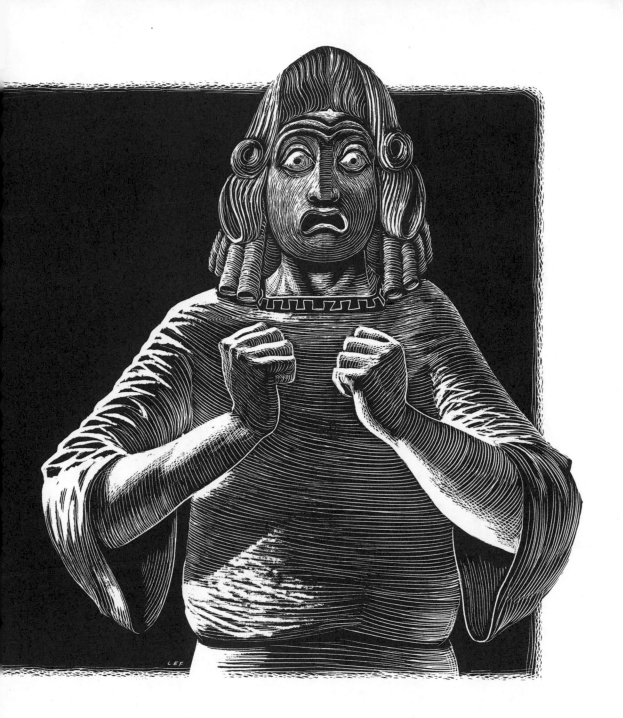

or not they were bald. The style was set by those nobles of King Louis' court who could afford to follow their monarch's lead. Suddenly everyone at court began to wear the most expensive and elaborate wigs that could be made.

The *HISTORY*

The custom continued in France throughout the reign of Louis XIV, who was also going bald. It was not until 1663, however, that wearing a wig became a really widespread fashion. In that year, Charles II, who had been restored to the throne of England after the reign of the Puritans, put on a large curly black wig to cover his graying hair. The whole English aristocracy followed his lead, as did those others who only wished to look aristocratic and fashionable.

The English called their hairy headpieces *perukes,* after the French *perruques.* They also called them *periwigs.* From this name came the shorter word, *wig.*

The many different styles of wigs for men and women depended on the social occasion for which they were to be worn, or on the profession, service, and trade of the wearer. Most of the wigs were worn by men. If the wearers were not bald

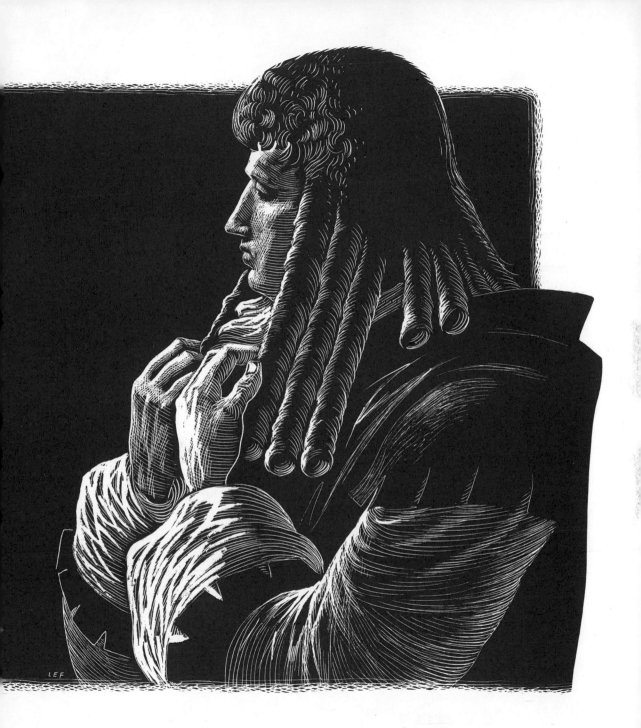

Some of the wigs
(Others are shown opposite
the title page
and on page 21)

to begin with, they soon would be made so by
the constant use of these hot and often heavy
headpieces. Wigs became a necessity of fashion,
and no one who wished to be thought important
dared be without one.

The HISTORY

Early in the eighteenth century, soldiers wore
a wig with a long braid, tied at the top with a
large bow and at the bottom with a small bow.
It was called a *ramillie* (RAM-i-lee). Travelers
wore a long, flowing wig loosely curled and with
a twisted lock on each side and curls about the
forehead — called a *campaign wig*. Ordinary people wore a curled wig called a *Sunday buckle,* or
more often, a *major bob*. Apprentices and poor
people wore a *minor bob*, a wide bushy wig parted
down the center.

Among the more popular styles were the *bagwig,* with the long hairs at the back tied inside a
small silk bag; the *cadogan,* worn by outlandishly
dressed young dandies; and the *square,* worn by
judges and the nobility. There were also wigs
called the *vallancy,* with long flowing curls; the
brigadier, a short length of hair, tied, with two
curls at the bottom; the double pigtail *queue;*
the *natural wig*; and the *knotted wig.*

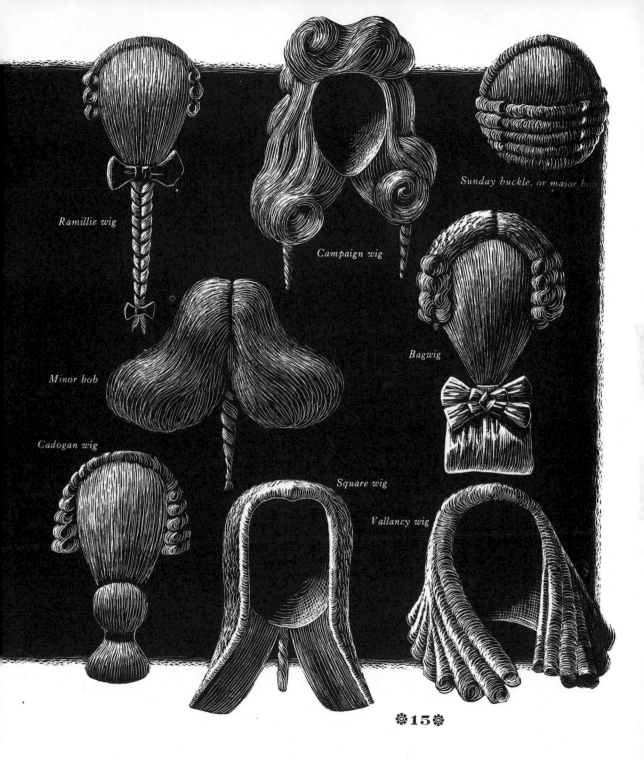

Ramillie wig

Campaign wig

Sunday buckle, or major bob

Minor bob

Bagwig

Cadogan wig

Square wig

Vallancy wig

❂15❂

The craze for wig-wearing quickly spread to America, where newly arrived aristocrats and the King's officials insisted on keeping up with fashion even in the wilderness.

The HISTORY

A great wave of protest by some members of the clergy and by Puritan officials soon broke over the heads of the wig-wearers, however. In 1675 the Massachusetts Court denounced wig-wearing men, and said they looked like women. The court chose to ignore the fact that the Governor of New Hampshire had been wearing a wig since 1670. Soon all New England was in an uproar. Many a Puritan preacher took to his pulpit to condemn the fashion as having "no warrant in the word of God." Other Puritan preachers, wearing wigs, rose in their pulpits to call down their fellow ministers for speaking "against an innocent fashion taken up and used by the best of men."

John Eliot, the Massachusetts missionary to the Indians, noted the calamities suffered by the colonists in their war with the Indians, known as King Philip's War. Eliot was certain that the trouble was a punishment from God for wig-wearing.

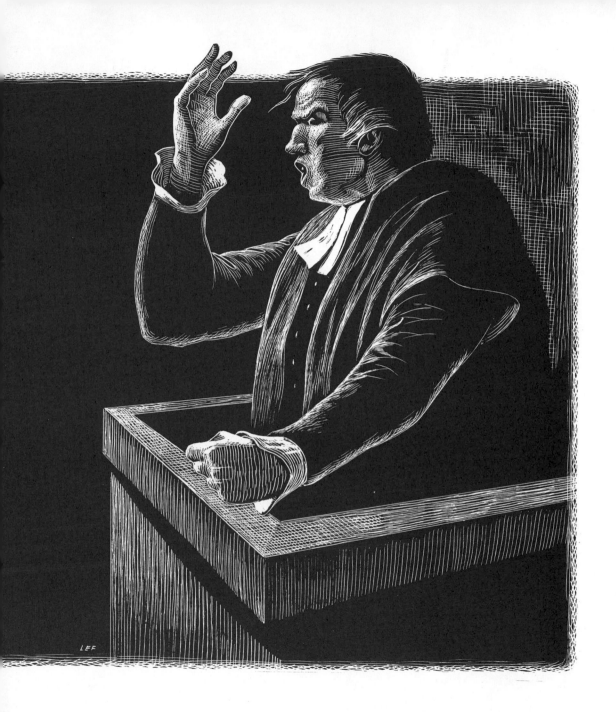

The *HISTORY*

Increase Mather, the famous Puritan minister of Boston, raged against wigs, calling them "horrid bushes of vanity." But his own son, Cotton Mather, delighted in wearing one of these "bushes." The students at Harvard College took to wig-wearing, while the president of the college worried about it and warned against it. Judge Samuel Sewall of Boston would not attend a church service conducted by a wig-wearing parson.

None of the abuse heaped on the wig-wearers halted the fashion. If anything, it spurred everyone, including the clergy, to continue wearing wigs.

The southern colonies had no such problem as Massachusetts had. Wealthy Virginian planters and gentlemen, as well as blacksmiths, innkeepers, bricklayers, and clergymen, all wore wigs. Only the poor rural farmers did not wear them.

The wealthy colonists usually ordered their most expensive wigs from London, while the not-so-wealthy had theirs made by local barbers and wigmakers. Wigmaking in America became such good business that many a London craftsman left

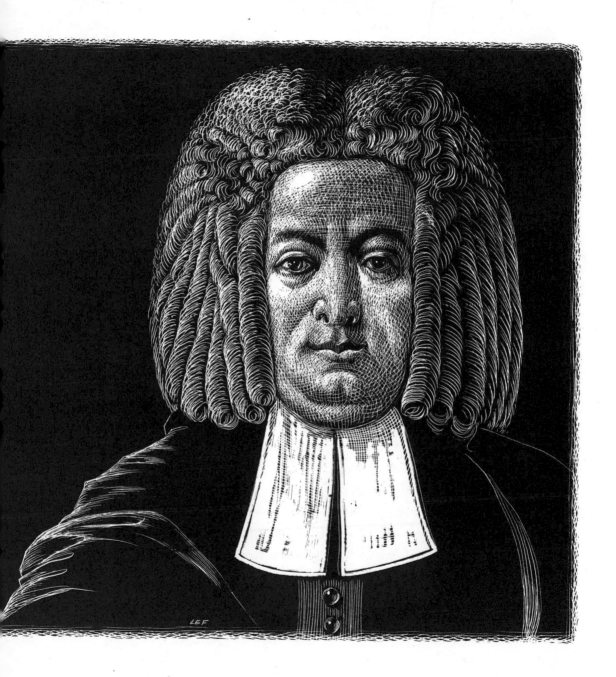

England and established himself in the colonies. In the Virginia capital of Williamsburg in 1769 there were at least eight wigmaking craftsmen busily engaged in their work. All in all, some thirty wigmakers worked in that small city between 1700 and 1780.

The HISTORY

Few wigmakers anywhere in the colonies were without orders for making new wigs or sprucing up worn ones. It seemed as if no one wanted to be seen wearing his natural hair, however much of it he might have. Wigmakers were rewarded in praise and money for keeping up the high quality of workmanship needed to please their vain and fashion-crazy public.

After the War for Independence had been won, however, the wigmaking business in America slowly grew smaller. A new era was beginning, and new eras bring new fashions with them. Once again all eyes turned to France, for in 1789 the Parisians began their own revolution against the monarchy — and started a new democratic way of life in which wig-wearing had no part.

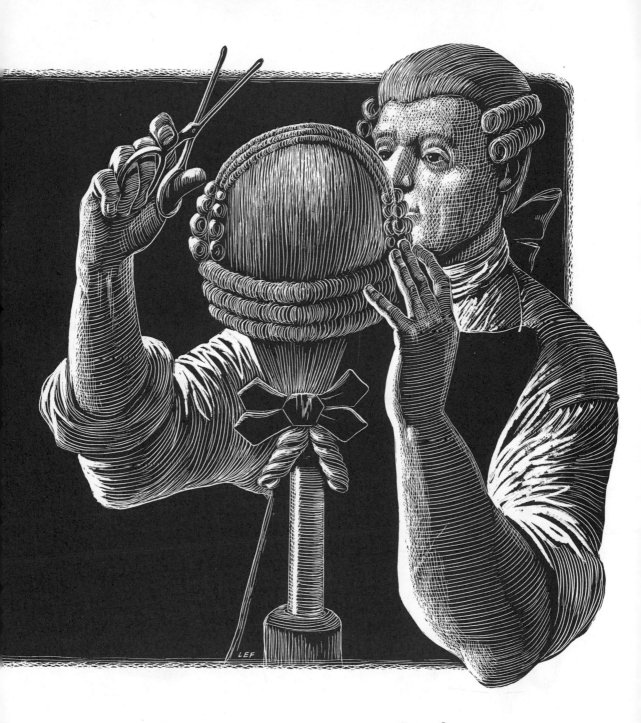

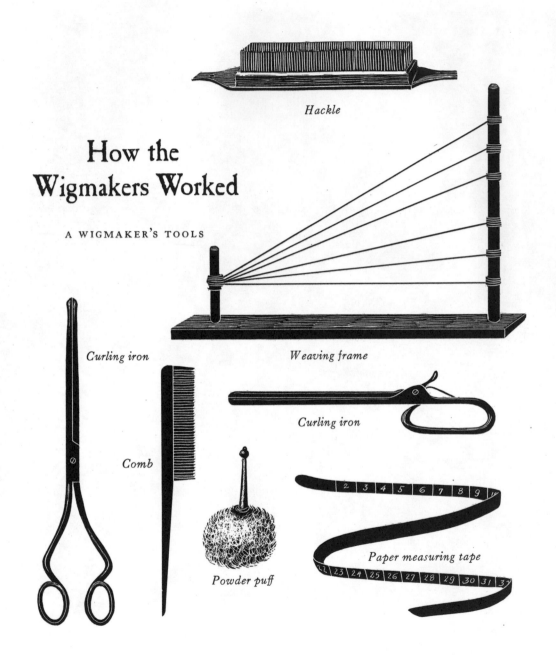

Hackle

How the Wigmakers Worked

A WIGMAKER'S TOOLS

Curling iron

Weaving frame

Curling iron

Comb

Powder puff

Paper measuring tape

FEW WIGS WERE BOUGHT READY MADE. Each was usually fashioned especially to fit the person who was to wear it. The wigmaker could make any one of more than a hundred different styles and he could use any one of a variety of colors. In colors, there was a choice of brown, pale yellow, chestnut, auburn, gray, white, black, and a mixture of these last two, called grizzle. It remained for the customer to decide what style and color suited him best.

Once that was decided, the wigmaker, who was usually a barber, too, shaved his customer's head to prepare it for measurement.

The head was measured by using narrow strips of paper that marked off five distances:

from the center of the forehead to the nape of the neck across the top of the head,

from the right temple to the left temple around the back of the head,

from ear to ear, across the top of the head,

from the center of the forehead to the left and right temples,

from each cheek to the back of the head.

The *TECHNIQUE*

☼ 23 ☼

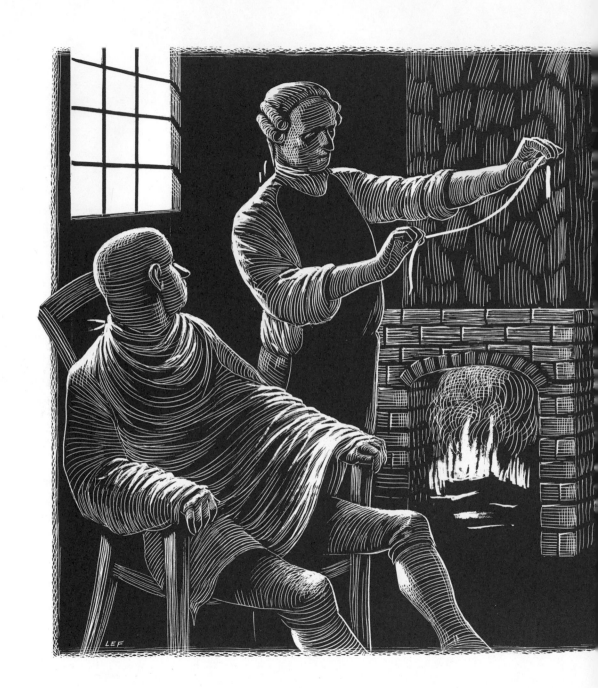

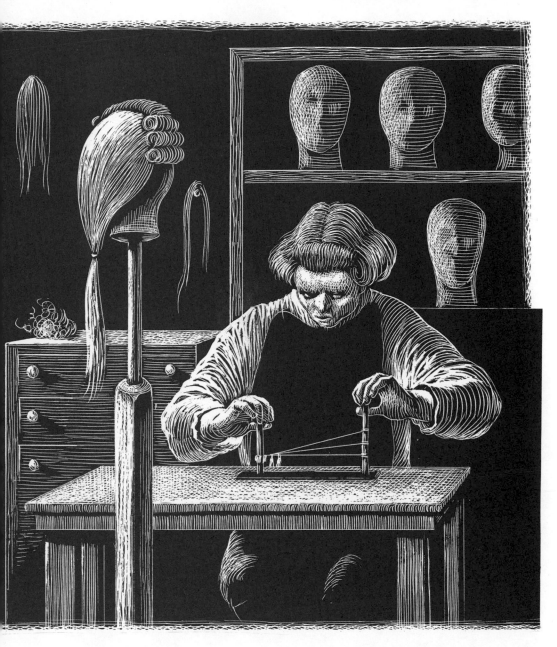

A wigmaker's shop

The *TECHNIQUE*

Once the measuring had been done, the customer put on his old wig or, if he had none as yet, covered his shaven head with a skullcap, fancy turban, or hood, and went home. He was not needed again except to call for his finished wig, try it on, and pay for it.

The wigmaker now began to prepare the hair for the wig. Much of the hair used in the colonies was imported from England by hair merchants. Some of it was already prepared. Only the finest quality of human hair was used. More often than not, women's hair was found to be stronger than that of men. The hair of a country woman was considered better than that of a woman who lived in the city.

In preparing the hair, it was tied in small bundles, or *parcels,* and cleaned with flour dust and fine sand to rid it of its natural oils. The parcel of hair was then pulled through a comb called a *hackle,* and was separated and rearranged in parcels of varying lengths, thicknesses, and colors. Each parcel was next held in a vise while the strand of hair was rolled around a clay curling pin. When all the parcels had been rolled, the

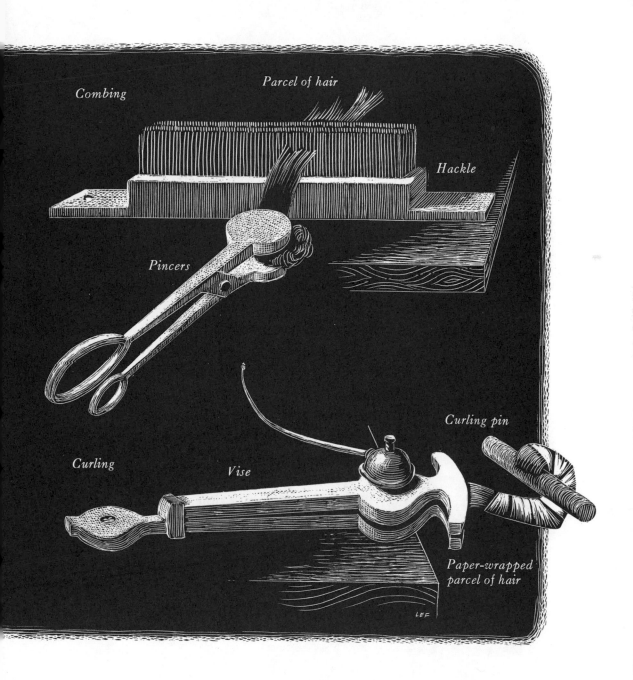

Combing

Parcel of hair

Hackle

Pincers

Curling

Curling pin

Vise

Paper-wrapped
parcel of hair

LEF

☼ 27 ☼

curling pins were boiled, and dried in a small, cylindrical oven. They were then taken to a bakery, where they were covered with rye dough and baked.

Once baked, the *loaves* of curled hair were brought back to the wigmaker, who cut them apart. The baked curls, still slightly moist from the dough, were removed, and returned to the small, round oven for a final drying. When completely dry, they were slipped from their clay pins, combed again through the hackle, checked for strength, fullness, and color, and were then trimmed.

All these preparations were necessary to *temper* the hair: that is, give it strength and flexibility. Tempering not only made the hair workable for the craftsman, but also made it durable, so that the wig lasted a long time.

The wigmaker next looked at a pattern showing the length and arrangement of hairs in the style of wig he wished to make. He then drew a set of parallel lines on a sheet of paper already marked off in squares. These parallel lines formed a pattern that followed the measurements he had

The *TECHNIQUE*

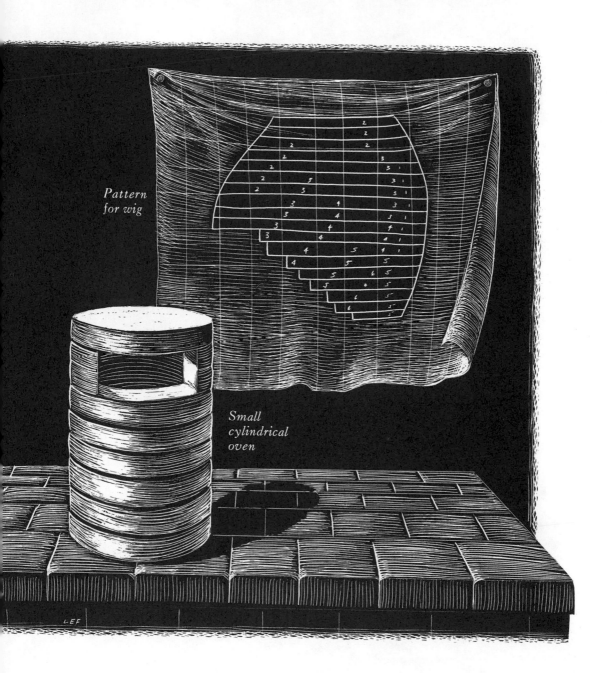

Pattern
for wig

Small
cylindrical
oven

LEF

The *TECHNIQUE*

made on the customer's head with the narrow paper strips. All the lines together made a plan of the customer's head, which the wig was to cover. On each line the wigmaker noted the length of hair to be used in that particular portion of the wig.

With his marked-off plan he now sat down at a table that held a *weaving frame.* The weaving frame was made up of three or six silk threads tightly stretched between two vertical pegs. Three threads on the frame represented one side of the wig. Six threads on the frame represented both sides of the wig. The upper three were the left side. The lower three were the right side.

The wigmaker picked up several strands of hair and began weaving them in and out and up and down around the silk threads of the frame. Thus he fastened the strands of hair in place, while leaving their curled ends free.

When a few strands had been woven according to the measurements shown in the pattern, he slid them tightly together into a strip. These woven hairs were called the *weft.* After a strip of weft had been finished, the wigmaker turned one

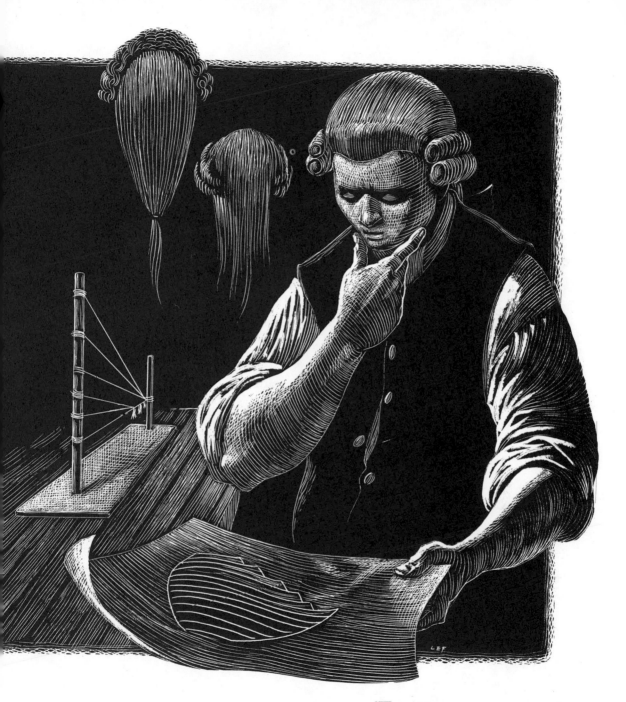

The **TECHNIQUE**

of the pegs of the weaving frame, winding the strip around it while at the same time more silk thread was unwound from the other peg. With this thread the weaver started a new strip. He continued to weave and wind until he had all the strips of weft called for by the pattern.

The next step was to make a support, or *caul*, that would fit on the head and hold the hairs. To do this, the wigmaker placed a wooden *wig block* on a stand. The wig block was roughly the same size and shape as the customer's head, as shown by the five measurements. Silk ribbons an inch wide, called *mounting ribbon,* were fitted onto the block in the exact head outline of the wig that was being made. The ribbons were sewn together, and tightly fixed to the wig block by threading them to a row of nails called *wig points.*

When the mounting ribbons had been fastened firmly and exactly in place, the wigmaker sewed a fine silk net to them. Over this he put two wide bands of *covering ribbon.* One band stretched across the top of the block from front to back. The other band stretched across the top from side to side. With this done, the wigmaker added

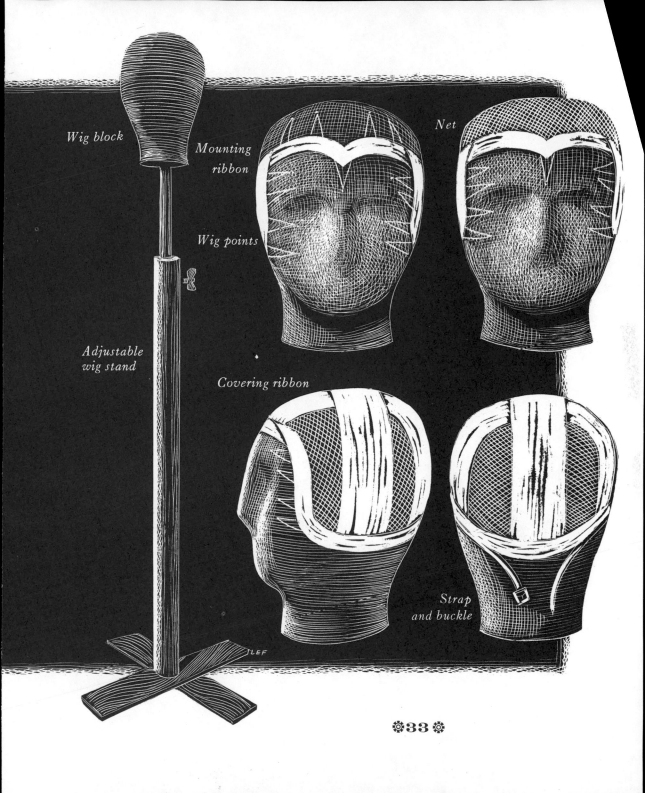

Wig block

Mounting ribbon

Net

Wig points

Adjustable wig stand

Covering ribbon

Strap and buckle

❁33❁

a strap and buckle or a drawstring at the back of the caul. By using this, the customer could fasten his wig as tightly as he pleased.

Next, the wigmaker sewed the strips of woven hair, or weft, to the caul. He was always careful to follow the pattern for the length of hairs and rows, so that he would end up with the style of wig the customer had ordered. Usually the wigmaker began sewing at the bottom back of the caul and gradually worked to the top and front. The rows of hairs that framed the face of the customer were the only ones that were sewn at the front edge of the caul and worked toward the back.

The *TECHNIQUE*

When all the strips of weft had been sewn in place, the wig was ready to be *finished* and *dressed.*

Finishing called for the greatest skill. Each curl must be gracefully rounded, and the straight parts must be combed to perfection. With a curling iron, comb, scissors, and his fingers, the wigmaker carefully shaped and trimmed every part of the wig.

As last touches, silk bags or ribbon ties were

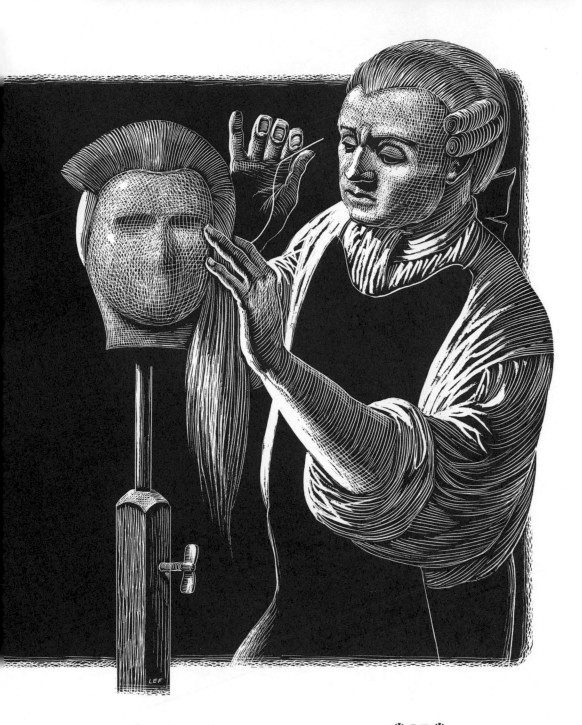

*The final fitting
of the wig
to the customer*

added at the back, according to the style. The wig was then sprayed with perfume, and powdered in a tone that matched the color of the hairpiece. These final steps were called dressing.

The *TECHNIQUE*

When the dressing was completed, the customer was notified. He returned to the wigmaker's shop for a fitting. If everything had been done to his satisfaction, he paid for his wig and either wore it out of the shop or carried it home in a specially built wig box.

The wigmaker's work was never quite done, however. Wigs had to be constantly cared for. Powder and perfume quickly lost their effect. Curls came undone, and straight hairs uncombed. The wigmaker was hired by the month or the year to keep his handiwork in top condition. He did this as a traveling service, going from house to house. For special occasions such as Saturday evening social events, wigs were brought to the shop, where they were freshened and returned to the owner. On a Saturday afternoon it was not unusual to see scores of wigmakers' apprentices dashing through the narrow streets of Boston or any other early American city, rushing to deliver

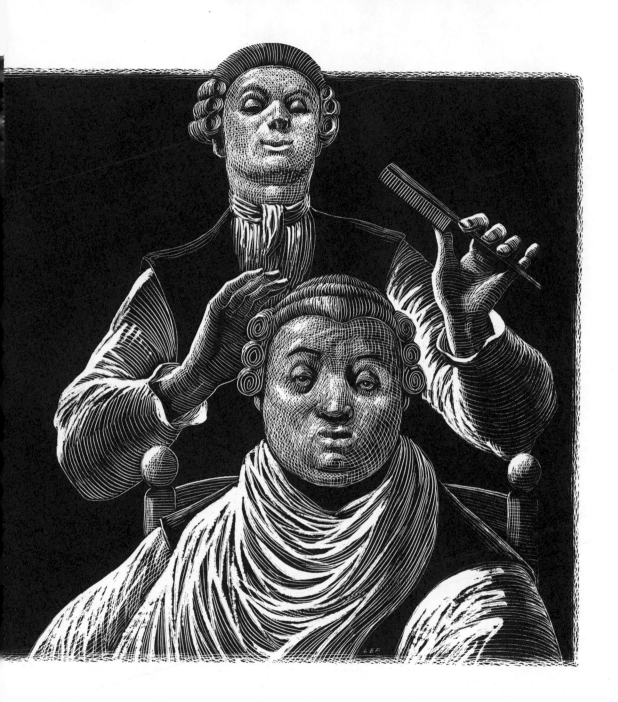

*Apprentices delivered
freshly curled and
powdered wigs in wig boxes*

The *TECHNIQUE*

the freshly curled and powdered wigs belonging to the great and near-great men of the day.

The careful workmanship of the wigmaker was demanded of him by colonial people who took pride in their appearance. It was the pride of those who valued their place in the life of a new and promising nation. &

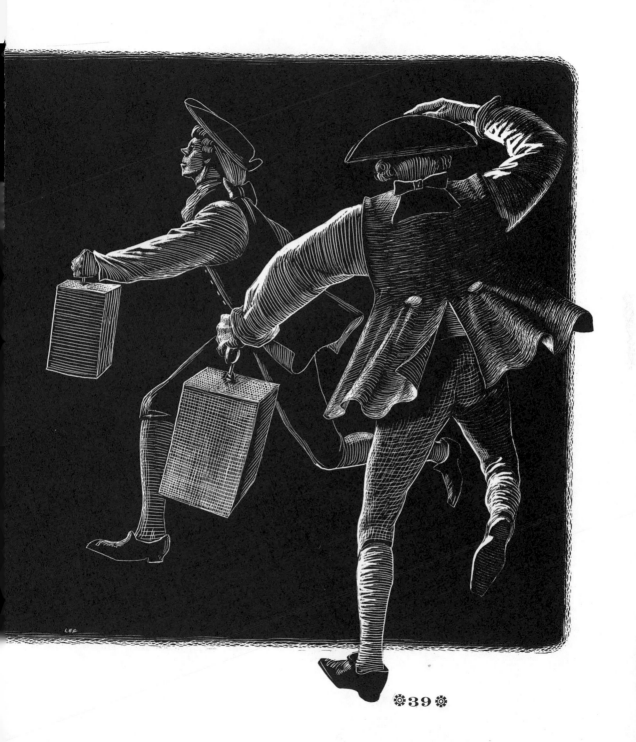

Wigmakers' Terms

BAGWIG — A wig with the long hairs at the back tied inside a small silk bag.

BRIGADIER — A type of wig cut in a short lock, with two curls at the bottom.

CADOGAN — A type of wig that was formerly worn by extremely dressed young dandies.

CAMPAIGN WIG — A type of wig worn for traveling, with a twisted lock on each side and curls about the forehead.

CAUL — The ribbon and net foundation for a wig.

COVERING RIBBON — The two wide bands of ribbon — one stretching from front to back, one from side to side — that were part of the caul.

DRESSING — The spraying, powdering, and adding of decorative touches that were the final steps in wigmaking.

FINISHING — The final combing, curling, shaping, and trimming of the wig.

HACKLE — The comb through which hair was passed in preparing it for the wig.

LOAVES — The baked curls of hair for the wig, with their covering of dough.

MAJOR BOB — A type of curled wig, sometimes called a Sunday buckle.

MINOR BOB — A wide, bushy wig, parted down the center.

MOUNTING RIBBON — A foundation of ribbon for the wig, arranged to fit the head; part of the caul.

PARCELS — The strands of hair, separated into small

bundles for baking and curling in preparation for wig-making.

PERIWIG — An English term for the French *perruque,* or wig.

Perruque — The French term for a wig.

PERUKE — An English term for the French *perruque,* or wig.

QUEUE — A type of wig with braids hanging down the back.

RAMILLIE — A type of wig with a long braid, tied at top and bottom with bows.

SQUARE WIG — A type of wig worn by judges and the nobility.

SUNDAY BUCKLE — A type of curled wig, more often called a major bob.

TEMPERING — The cleaning, curling, and baking of the hair, in preparation for wigmaking.

VALLANCY — A type of wig with long, flowing curls.

WEAVING FRAME — A frame holding silk threads, on which the hair was woven into strips for the wig.

WEFT — A strip of hair woven to form part of a wig.

WIG BLOCK — The head-shaped block on which the caul and wig were fashioned according to proper measurements for each customer.

WIG POINTS — Little nails in the wig block which held the caul in place while the wigmaker worked.

Index

Artist Leonard Everett Fisher says this of his books on early American craft workers: "I chose to write and illustrate a group of books on colonial American craftsmen because I know of no other time in our history when the aspirations of the people were so clearly expressed by their extraordinary craftsmanship. They were artists in every sense of the word. Their skill was a matter of profound and lengthy training. They applied themselves with energy and care. Their attitude was always one of pride in their singular ability and individualism. They were deliberate workmen who exercised such great control over their ideas, tools, and materials that they created one-of-a-kind objects that could not be recreated. The craftsman was master of his creations.

"I want my children to know this. I want their friends to know this. It is a most meaningful part of their history."

Mr. Fisher is a graduate of Yale Art School, where he was awarded the Weir Prize, the Winchester Fellowship, and an appointment as Assistant in Design Theory. Well known as an artist and an illustrator of children's books, as well as an author, his outstanding graphic work has been recognized by the American Institute of Graphic Arts in its exhibits of Outstanding Textbooks and Outstanding Children's Books.

The text of this book has been composed on the linotype in Caslon 137. This face is derived from the great oldstyle cut by William Caslon of London in the early eighteenth century. Caslon types were used widely by American printers during the colonial period and even today it is considered to be "the finest vehicle for the conveyance of English speech that the art of the punch-cutter has yet devised."

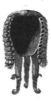

Natural Norwood Offset paper
supplied by Tileston & Hollingsworth Company, Boston

Composed by Lettick Typografic, Bridgeport

Printed by The Moffa Press, Inc., New York

Bound by H. Wolff Book Manufacturing Company, Inc., New York

DESIGNED BY BERNARD KLEIN